Your Diet
INFLAMMATION
&
YOUR HEALTH

PRINCE N. AGBEDANU, PhD

Book Design: Nonon Tech & Design

ISBN: 978-1-959642-02-2 (Paperback)

Table of Contents

Introduction

In this ebook, we'll discuss Inflammation and how it's related to the spinal nerves. We'll also touch on the different types of Inflammation, as well as the mechanism of Inflammation. Finally, we'll answer the question, "Why do spinal nerves suffer the most effect from inflammation?"

Inflammation is a reaction of the body to stimuli that can be either physical or chemical in nature. The purpose of this response is to protect tissues by removing harmful agents and initiating repair processes. However, when Inflammation persists for prolonged periods of time, it can lead to tissue damage and disease.

There are two main types of Inflammation: acute and chronic. Acute Inflammation is a short-lived response that occurs in response to injury or infection. On the other hand, chronic inflammation is a long-term response that can last for months or even years.

The mechanism of Inflammation involves the release of inflammatory mediators from immune cells. These mediators include histamine, prostaglandins, and leukotrienes. These substances cause blood vessels to dilate and increase permeability, which allows white blood cells and fluids to enter the affected tissues.

One of the most common sites of chronic Inflammation is the spine. This is because the spinal nerves are constantly exposed to potentially harmful agents, such as bacteria and viruses. In addition, the spine is also subject to physical stressors, such as repetitive motion and poor posture. All of these factors can contribute to developing chronic Inflammation of the spine.

If you're suffering from chronic Inflammation of the spine, it's essential to seek treatment. Treatment options include anti-inflammatory medications, physical therapy, and surgery. A combination of these treatments may sometimes be necessary to achieve relief.

If you're looking for more information on Inflammation and its relationship to the spine, read our complete ebook. In it, we'll cover everything you need to know about this topic, including the different types of Inflammation, the mechanism of Inflammation, and why spinal nerves are particularly susceptible to its effects.

PART I:

CHAPTER 1

An introduction to Inflammation

I t is a process that occurs when your body's white blood cells and their chemicals protect you from infection or injury. In some cases, Inflammation can be beneficial – for example, when it helps heal a cut or wound. But long-term inflammation can damage your body and leads to disease [1].

The two types of inflammation are namely acute and chronic. Acute inflammation is a normal response to injury or infection; it typically goes away once the threat is eliminated. But when inflammation becomes chronic, it can last for months or even years, contributing to deleterious chronic diseases like heart disease, cancer, and arthritis.

INFLAMMATION PATHWAY

The inflammatory response is a complex biological process that helps the body to remove potential threats and heal tissue damage. Four main steps characterize it: capillary widening, increased permeability of capillaries, the attraction of leukocytes, and systemic response (figure 1).

The process of inflammation following tissue injury

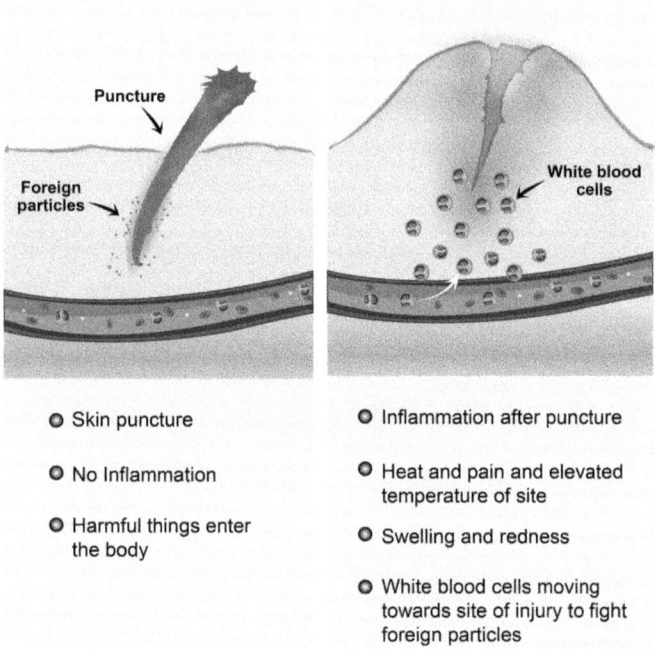

○ Skin puncture	○ Inflammation after puncture
○ No Inflammation	○ Heat and pain and elevated temperature of site
○ Harmful things enter the body	○ Swelling and redness
	○ White blood cells moving towards site of injury to fight foreign particles

Figure 1: The process of inflammation following tissue injury.

THE PROCESS OF INFLAMMATION FOLLOWING TISSUE INJURY

1. Capillary Widening: When an injury or infection occurs, the body responds by dilating (widening) the blood vessels in the affected area. This allows more blood to flow to the site of injury or infection and helps deliver adequate oxygen and nutrients for healing.

2. Increased Permeability of Capillaries: In addition to widening, the walls of the blood vessels also become more permeable, allowing plasma and leukocytes (white blood cells) to leak out into the tissues, where they can assist in the healing process.

3. Attraction of Leukocytes: Once in the tissues, leukocytes are attracted to the site of injury or infection by various chemical signals.

4. Systemic Response: The inflammatory response also triggers a systemic response in the whole body, which releases hormones to boost the immune system and enhance the healing process.

MECHANISMS INVOLVED IN INFLAMMATION

Hence, what causes inflammation to become chronic? The answer lies in the mechanisms involved in inflammation. There are three primary mechanisms involved in inflammation: cellular activation, cytokine production, and chemokine signaling [1]. These mechanisms play a critical role in developing chronic diseases [2]. So, let us take a detailed look at each one.

CELLULAR ACTIVATION

Cellular activation is the process by which body cells become activated in response to an injury or infection. It begins with the detection of the threat by the white blood cells. After this, they release chemicals known as cytokines. These cytokines signal other cells to enter the site of injury or infection [3].

This influx of cells leads to an "inflammatory response." This response is characterized by redness, swelling, and heat. While these symptoms may be beneficial in the short term, they can cause damage to your body if they stay for an extended period [4].

CYTOKINE PRODUCTION

Cytokines are proteins released by your body's cells in response to an injury or infection. They help regulate the immune response, and they also play a role in inflammation.

There are two types of cytokines: pro-inflammatory and anti-inflammatory. Pro-inflammatory cytokines promote the early stages of inflammation, while anti-inflammatory cytokines help resolve it. When your body's cells produce too many pro-inflammatory cytokines, it leads to chronic inflammation and the development of diseases [5].

CHEMOKINE SIGNALING

Chemokines are proteins that help regulate the movement of cells. They do this by binding to receptors on the surface of cells and signaling them to move towards or away from specific areas.

Some chemokines are pro-inflammatory, while others are anti-inflammatory. Pro-inflammatory chemokines include CCL2, CCL3, and CCL5. These chemokines are involved in the movement of immune cells toward areas of inflammation. They also activate the white blood cells once they arrive at the site of inflammation. Anti-inflammatory chemokines include CCL4 and CCL8. These chemokines help reduce inflammation by promoting the movement of immune cells away from areas of inflammation [1].

Chemokine signaling is a complex process that is not fully understood. However, the balance of pro- and anti-inflammatory chemokines is essential for maintaining healthy inflammation levels.

CHAPTER 2

The Mediators of Inflammation: Eicosanoids

Eicosanoids are lipid mediators that play a role in the regulation of inflammation. There are three main types of eicosanoids: prostaglandins, leukotrienes, and thromboxanes, which play distinct roles in regulating inflammation [6].

As the human body responds to injury or infection, inflammation is crucial. However, inflammation can induce diseases, such as autoimmune diseases, allergies, and cancer, when inflammation goes unregulated [5]. Eicosanoids help offset such conditions. They help regulate the inflammatory response by promoting blood flow to the injury site and inhibiting the release of inflammatory mediators. In other words, they aid in keeping inflammation in check.

All three eicosanoids play an essential role in the inflammatory process. However, they each have different functions and effects on the body. So, let's take a closer look at each one.

First, we have prostaglandins. Prostaglandins are hormones that enhance the blood flow to the injury site by causing vasodilation or widening of the blood vessels [7]. This increased blood flow allows more nutrients and oxygen to reach the injured area, which aids in healing. Additionally, prostaglandins reduce inflammation by inhibiting the release of other inflammatory mediators like histamine and leukotrienes. Prostaglandins also have undesirable effects. For example, they dilate the blood vessels in the forehead and brain, which causes a headache, specifically migraine [8]. A group of non-steroidal anti-inflammatory drugs (NSAIDS) can block the production of prostaglandins and are useful for treating headaches. You are likely aware of the most used NSAID, known as aspirin, which you must have taken at some stage of your life to treat headaches [9].

Next, we have leukotrienes. Leukotrienes are chemicals that promote vasoconstriction by reducing the diameter of the blood vessels. The reduced blood flow means reduced delivery of nutrients and oxygen to the injury site. Leukotrienes also stimulate the release of other inflammatory mediators like histamine and prostaglandins [10]. Leukotrienes are essential for developing inflammatory diseases such as asthma and allergies [4].

Finally, we have thromboxanes, which are chemicals that promote platelet aggregation and vasoconstriction by narrowing the blood vessels. These eicosanoids are produced by platelets and have pro-inflammatory effects. In other words, thromboxanes can be considered "bad" eicosanoids because they promote inflammation.

All three of these mediators play critical roles in regulating inflammation; however, they have different effects on the human body depending on their concentration levels. When all three mediators are present in high concentrations, they can amplify each other's products and lead to severe tissue damage. However, when all three mediators are present in low concentrations, they can balance each other out and lead to improved healing. Therefore, it is vital to maintain a balance of all three mediators to minimize tissue damage during injury or illness.

THE TRIGGERS OF EICOSANOID PRODUCTION

Different triggers can cause eicosanoid production. These triggers include injury, infection, inflammation, allergens, and stress [7]. When any of these triggers are present, they can cause an increase in the production of eicosanoids, which can lead to various effects on the body, depending on the type of eicosanoid produced.

Tissue injury is a common trigger for eicosanoid production. When you injure yourself, your body responds by increasing blood flow to the injury site, which causes an increase in the production of prostaglandins and thromboxanes. Additionally, the release of other inflammatory mediators like histamine and leukotrienes is also increased. This increased eicosanoid production can lead to increased inflammation, tissue damage, and pain.

Infection is another trigger that can cause eicosanoid production. When you are infected with bacteria or viruses, your body responds by increasing white blood cell activity at the site of infection. This leads to an increase in the production of leukotrienes and prostaglandins. These eicosanoids help fight off the infection by increasing blood flow to the site and promoting inflammation [11].

Stress is another trigger that can cause eicosanoid production [10]. When you are under stress, your body releases cortisol, which is an eicosanoid that helps prepare your body for the "fight or flight" response. This eicosanoid increases blood flow to your muscles, heart, and lungs and suppresses immunity. Conversely, it reduces blood flow to your intestines and stomach. Allergens may also induce the production of eicosanoids.

For example, your body produces histamine in response to an allergen, which helps to protect your body from the irritant by causing inflammation.

Changes in temperature or humidity levels also trigger eicosanoid production. For example, exposure to cold weather can cause the release of leukotrienes, which help keep the body warm by constricting blood vessels in the skin and increasing the body's metabolic rate. Exposure to hot weather can cause the release of prostaglandins, which help to protect the body from overheating by sweating. Changes in humidity can also trigger eicosanoid production; for example, dry air triggers the release of leukotrienes, which help moisturize the airways by increasing mucus production.

FOOD TRIGGERS OF INFLAMMATION

There is no one-size-fits-all answer to this usual question, as the foods that trigger inflammation can vary from person to person. However, some common culprits tend to trigger inflammation in many people (figure 2). These include sugary enriched and processed foods, as well as foods that are high in saturated or trans fats, including oily and fried stuff [12]. Additionally, certain foods may irritate the digestive system, leading to inflammation. Common offenders include dairy products, gluten-containing foods, and spicy foods [13].

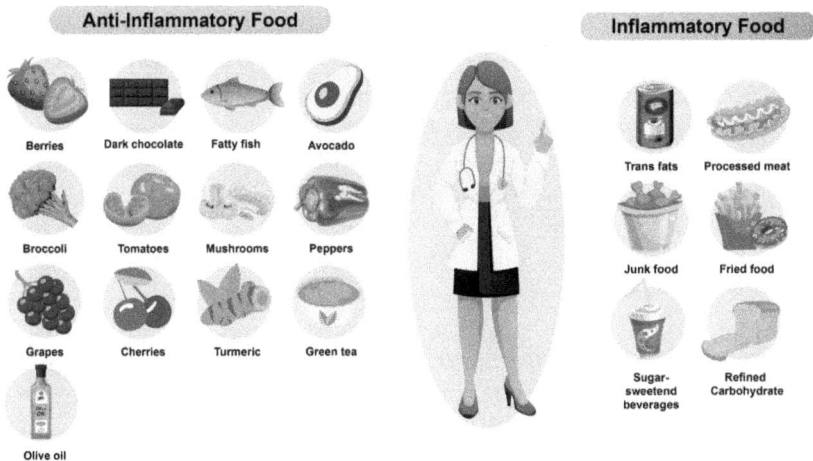

Figure 2: Foods that promote inflammation.

FOODS THAT PROMOTE INFLAMMATION INCLUDE:

sugar-sweetened beverages, refined carbohydrates, fried foods, trans fat and processed meat.

There is no denying that sugar is delicious to many people. But it is also one of the worst culprits in triggering inflammation. That's because sugar promotes the release of inflammatory cytokines and increases oxidative stress or the production of free radicals in the body [14]. So, if you are trying to keep inflammation at bay, it's best to cut back on sweets.

Refined carbohydrates are pro-inflammatory, just like sugar. They are broken down into simple sugars, and can lead to a sudden spike in blood sugar levels, which triggers an inflammatory response. So, if you want to reduce inflammation, limiting your intake of refined carbs such as white bread, pasta, and pastries is the best.

Trans fats are created when manufacturers add hydrogen to vegetable oils to make them solid at room temperature (think: margarine and shortening). Trans-fats promote inflammation by increasing oxidative stress and LDL cholesterol levels—and they've been linked to increased heart disease and the chances of stroke. To avoid trans fats, avoid fried foods, processed foods, and anything else that contains partially hydrogenated oils.

Saturated fats are another common type of fat that triggers inflammation [12]. They're found in animal-based foods such as red meat, full-fat dairy, and eggs. Saturated fats can increase low-density-lipoproteins cholesterol (LDL) or harmful cholesterol levels and promote plaque formation in the arteries— a common risk factor for heart disease and stroke.

Moderate alcohol consumption is often considered healthy. But when it comes to inflammation, even average daily alcohol intake can negatively affect health. That's because alcohol increases oxidative stress and impairs immunity. So, it's best to constrain your alcohol intake or avoid it altogether. Instead, opt for non-alcoholic beverages like water or herbal tea.

Omega-6 fatty acids are mandatory for our health, but too much can promote inflammation [15]. This is because they compete with omega-3 fatty acids for space in our cells. When there's an imbalance between omega-3 and omega-6 fatty acids levels, pro-inflammatory substances are produced, leading to inflammation. To avoid this problem, ensure you're getting an adequate amount of omega-3 fatty acids in your diet and limit your intakes of inflammatory omega-6 fatty acids, like vegetable oils and processed meats.

It's no secret that dairy products can be hard to digest, particularly for lactose-intolerant people. But even if you don't have any trouble digesting milk or cheese, they can still cause inflammation in your gut [14]. This is because dairy products are enriched in a type of sugar called lactose, which can be difficult for your body to break down. Additionally, many dairy products are high in saturated fat, a typical inflammation trigger. If you find that dairy gives you digestive problems, try cutting back or eliminating it from your diet altogether.

If you have celiac disease or are gluten-sensitive, you already know that you must avoid gluten. But even if you don't have an allergy or sensitivity to gluten, it can still irritate your digestive system. Gluten is a protein found in wheat, rye, and barley. When it meets the lining of your gut, it can cause inflammation.

Spicy foods are a common trigger for digestive problems like heartburn and indigestion. But they can also cause inflammation in the gut. That's because spicy foods contain compounds that can irritate the lining of your digestive tract, which releases eicosanoids and promotes inflammation.

No one food is going to cause inflammation in everyone. But some common triggers tend to cause problems for many people. If you have chronic inflammation in your body, try cutting back on sugar, refined carbs, trans fats, saturated fats, alcohol, and spicy foods [16]. You may also want to limit your intake of dairy products, gluten-containing foods, and omega-6 fatty acids. Everyone is different, so experiment to see what works for you. And remember, if you have any allergies or sensitivities to certain foods, be sure to avoid those foods as well.

OTHER KEY AGENTS OF INFLAMMATION

In addition to diet, other vital agents of inflammation can contribute to health problems. These include smoking, stress, obesity, and exposure to environmental pollutants [17].

Chronic stress can negatively affect our health, both physically and psychologically. Physically, stress can lead to inflammation throughout the body, overriding the normal processes that help to keep us healthy. This can make us vulnerable to diseases like heart disease, infertility, brain diseases, and cancer [15, 18, 19]. Additionally, psychological stress can exacerbate inflammation through its impact on the immune system and fight-or-flight response [5]. In this sense, physical and mental stress are interrelated risk factors for inflammation and must be optimally managed to promote health and wellness.

Obesity is a significant public health concern, with one in three adults classed as obese. Furthermore, while most people are familiar with the physical health risks associated with obesity, less attention is paid to its role in promoting inflammation [13]. Fat cells are active tissue, producing inflammatory mediators circulating throughout the body. These circulating agents can promote low-grade systemic inflammation in all body parts, affecting physical and mental health. Chronic inflammation may also lead to a sedentary lifestyle, overeating, and weight gain over time. As such, managing obesity is not just about caring for one's physical health – it's about protecting against inflammation and promoting overall well-being [12].

Toxins like cigarette smoke, alcohol, and environmental pollutants can lead to inflammation [17]. These substances can damage cells and tissues, leading to the release of inflammatory mediators. This, in turn, sets off a chain reaction that can cause inflammation to persist long after the original insult has passed. This prolonged inflammation can be damaging and contribute to a wide range of diseases.

Allergens are a common trigger of inflammation. Exposure to pollen, pet dander, and certain foods can cause an inflammatory response in some people [12, 17]. This response is often characterized by swelling, redness, and itchiness. In severe cases, an allergic reaction can lead to a life-threatening emergency called anaphylaxis. Therefore, people who suffer from allergies need to be aware of their triggers and take steps to avoid them.

An imbalance of hormone levels, such as thyroid hormone, cortisol, and insulin, can lead to inflammation. This is because these hormones play a role in regulating the body's inflammatory response. When these hormones are out of balance, inflammation can persist even after the original cause has been removed. Therefore, people with hormone imbalances need to seek medical care and correct the imbalance through treatment.

So, as you can see, many different agents of inflammation can contribute to health problems. Therefore, managing these risk factors and creating a healthy lifestyle is vital to reduce your risk of inflammation-related diseases.

IMPLICATIONS OF INFLAMMATION

While inflammation is a necessary and natural process, chronic inflammation can have many negative implications for our health as it can introduce several diseases [10, 18, 20]. Chronic inflammation can also lead to weight gain. This is because inflammatory mediators can promote fat storage in the body. Additionally, fatigue is a common symptom of chronic inflammation. This fatigue can be both mental and physical, making it difficult to function daily.

Besides the implications for our physical health, inflammation can also severely impact our mental well-being. This is because the inflammatory response is a stress response. When we are constantly in a state of inflammation, our body is in a constant state of stress. This can lead to mental health problems like anxiety, depression, and other mental disorders [3, 5]. It can also affect our cognitive function and memory.

Thus, as you can observe, inflammation is a complex process that can have a range of negative implications for our health. It is therefore, mandatory to be aware of the risk factors for chronic inflammation and take steps to reduce them. This will help you protect your health and promote overall well-being.

INFLAMMATION AT CELLULAR LEVEL

Three primary types of blood cells regulate inflammatory response: neutrophils, macrophages, and lymphocytes. Each cell type plays a different role in the process.

For example, neutrophils are the first cells to arrive at the site of injury or infection. Their primary purpose is to establish a barrier between the damaged tissue and the rest of the body so that further damage does not occur. Once that barrier is in place, neutrophils release enzymes that break down bacteria and other foreign invaders. They have the ability to engulf or internalize foreign particles and are described as phagocytic.

Macrophages are larger than neutrophils, arriving on the scene a bit later [21]. Their primary job is to clean up any debris left behind by the neutrophils (e.g., dead bacteria, damaged tissue). They also release chemicals that help promote tissue repair.

Lymphocytes are a type of white blood cell that helps to regulate immunity. There are two primary types of lymphocytes: T cells and B cells. T cells kill infected cells, while B cells produce antibodies that help destroy bacteria, viruses, and more prominent pathogens. [1]. These antibodies are also helpful in remembering the invading pathogen for future disease attacks.

Besides these three primary types of cells, several other cells also play a role in the inflammatory response. These include mast cells, basophils, and eosinophils.

Mast cells are found in connective tissue and play a vital role in allergy and immunity. When they are activated, they release chemicals that develop inflammation. This can lead to various symptoms, including sneezing, watery eyes, and a runny nose. It can also cause hives, eczema, and asthma attacks.

Basophils are another essential type of white blood cell involved in the immune response to parasitic infections. They release chemicals that help kill the parasites. This can help to clear the infection and reduce the symptoms.

Eosinophils play a critical role in regulating the immune response to allergic reactions. They help release histamines, which are chemicals that cause the symptoms of an allergy, such as a runny nose or itchy skin. Eosinophils also help to fight off any infection that the allergic reaction may cause.

These are just a few of the numerous types of cells that play a vital role in the inflammatory response. Therefore, as you can see, it is a complex process involving many players.

THE EFFECTS OF INFLAMMATION

Now that we understand more about inflammation, let's answer the question: is inflammation necessarily harmful? The answer is: it depends on the condition and duration of inflammation.

Acute inflammation is a usual and necessary response to injury or infection. It helps to protect the body and promote healing. Without acute inflammation, we would be much more susceptible to illness and disease [1].

Chronic inflammation, on the other hand, is a different story. This is when the inflammatory response goes on for too long or is triggered by something that isn't an infection or injury (e.g., stress, pollution, unhealthy diet). Chronic inflammation frequently leads to various health problems and contributes to the symptoms of conditions like arthritis and asthma [2, 5, 22]. So, acute inflammation is not necessarily bad. However, chronic inflammation can be harmful to your health.

INFLAMMATION AT ORGAN LEVEL

Did you know that inflammation can affect different body parts in other ways? Some organs feel the most effect of inflammation. Let's take a closer look at these organs and how they are affected by inflammation.

The first organ that feels the most effective of inflammation is the liver. The liver filters toxins out of the blood and breaks down fats. When the liver is inflamed, it doesn't function well, and can't filter toxins as effectively. This can lead to a buildup of toxins in the blood and increased fat storage.

Inflammation in the brain has been linked to conditions like Alzheimer's disease, Parkinson's disease, multiple sclerosis, depression, and attention deficit hyperactivity disorder (ADHD) [5, 11, 15, 23]. These conditions can cause a wide range of symptoms, from mild problems with memory or movement to severe disability and even death.

The heart and cardiovascular system are also frequently affected by inflammation, which can induce conditions like coronary artery disease, heart failure, and stroke [2, 24]. Inflammation is considered an essential contributing factor to the development of these conditions.

Joint inflammation may lead to conditions like rheumatoid arthritis, osteoarthritis, and gout. These conditions can cause pain, stiffness, swelling, and joint damage. Finally, inflammation can also affect the lungs. Diseases like asthma, COPD, and lung cancer have all been linked to lung inflammation [4].

Inflammation is a usual and necessary response to injury or infection. However, chronic inflammation can be harmful to your health. Several organs are affected by chronic inflammation, including the liver, brain, heart, gut, joints, and lungs [4]. If you're dealing with chronic inflammation, you must talk to your doctor about ways to manage it. Some anti-inflammatory medications and lifestyle changes can help to reduce inflammation and improve your health.

CHAPTER 3

Common Symptoms of Inflammation

Inflammation is the body's natural response to injury or infection. It is a normal and healthy phase of the healing process. There are several symptoms of inflammation, but some of the most common are:

Heat: Inflammation often causes an area to feel warm to the touch. This is due to increased blood flow to the site.

Redness: The increased blood flow can also cause the skin to appear redder than usual.

Swelling: Inflammation can cause fluid to build up in the tissues, resulting in swelling of the injured area.

Pain: Inflammation often causes pain and tenderness by activating the pain sensor neurons.

Loss of function: Inflammation can make it challenging to move a joint or use a muscle.

You must see a doctor if you are experiencing any of these symptoms. They can determine if you have inflammation and recommend treatment. Treatment may include medication, physical therapy, or lifestyle changes.

DISEASES THAT RESULT FROM INFLAMMATION

We all know that inflammation is the root cause of many diseases, but did you know that quite a few disorders specifically result from inflammation? Here's a list of some of the most common ones (figure 3):

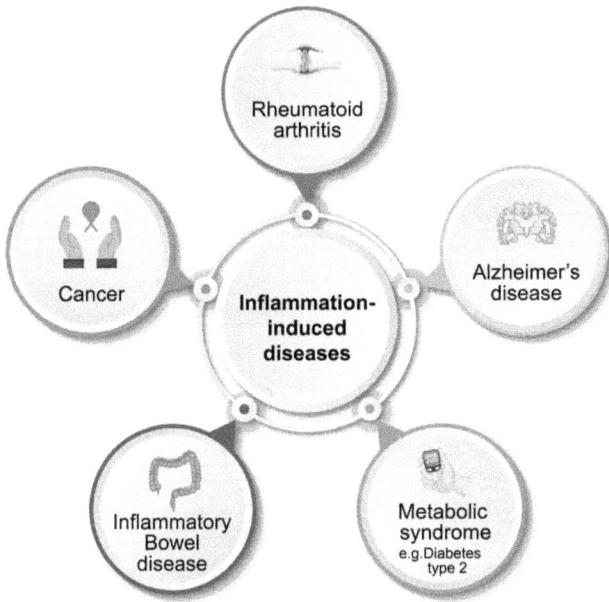

Figure 3: Diseases related to inflammation.

INFLAMMATION-INDUCED DISEASES INCLUDE:

Inflammatory bowel disease, metabolic syndrome related diseases such as the age onset type 2 diabetes mellitus, Rheumatoid arthritis, cancer and Alzheimer's disease.

Alzheimer's is a degenerative brain disorder resulting in memory loss, cognitive decline, and death. The disease is characterized by the buildup of plaques and tangles in the brain. While the exact cause of Alzheimer's disease is unknown, it is believed to be linked to inflammation. This is partly because patients with chronic inflammation are more susceptible to developing Alzheimer's disease [11].

Parkinson's disease is a neurodegenerative disorder that results in tremors, muscle stiffness, and difficulty maintaining balance and coordination. The disease is caused by the death of neurons in the brain that produce the neurotransmitter dopamine, which is partly due to inflammation of a local region [18].

Multiple sclerosis is an autoimmune disorder that attacks the central nervous system. The disease is characterized by inflammation of the myelin sheath, which protects nerve cells in a healthy individual. Multiple sclerosis can result in various symptoms, including muscle weakness, paralysis, and vision problems [4].

Rheumatoid arthritis is a chronic inflammatory disorder that affects the joints. The disease is characterized by swelling, pain, and stiffness of the joints of the hands. Rheumatoid arthritis can eventually lead to joint destruction and deformity with a dependent lifestyle [24].

Crohn's disease is a chronic inflammatory disorder that affects the digestive system. The disease is characterized by inflammation of the inner lining of the digestive tract, leading to abdominal pain, diarrhea, weight loss, and fatigue. Crohn's disease can also lead to severe complications such as intestinal blockages and malnutrition [2].

Heart disease is a general term used to describe various cardiovascular conditions. Heart disease is often caused by atherosclerosis, the buildup of plaque in the arteries. This plaque can lead to inflammation and blockages that can cause heart attacks and strokes [2].

Cancer is a group of diseases characterized by the uncontrolled growth of cells. Cancer can be caused by a variety of factors, including inflammation. Inflammation can damage DNA and lead to the formation of cancerous tumors [2].

Asthma is a chronic inflammatory disorder that affects the lungs. The disease is characterized by airway inflammation, leading to shortness of breath, wheezing, and coughing. Asthma can be triggered by various environmental factors, such as dust, pollen, or smoke.

Inflammation is a serious issue and will only become more of a problem as the population ages. Therefore, it is essential to know the inflammation symptoms and see a doctor if you are experiencing any of them. It's also important to be mindful of the diseases that can result from inflammation so that you can take steps to prevent them.

INFLAMMATION AND ATTENTION DEFICIT DISORDER (ADHD)

There is growing evidence that inflammation may play a role in developing ADHD [25]. One theory is that chronic inflammation may damage the executive function regions of the brain. These regions are responsible for planning, organizing, and paying attention. Another approach is that chronic inflammation may increase the level of certain neurotransmitters in the brain that play a role in ADHD [25].

There are no specific foods that individuals with ADHD must avoid. However, these individuals must eat a healthy and balanced diet [20]. A healthy diet includes plenty of fruits, vegetables, whole grains, and lean protein. Avoiding processed foods and sugary drinks [26]. These foods can trigger inflammation and may worsen ADHD symptoms.

If you or your child has ADHD, there are multiple things you can to try to help reduce inflammation. These include eating a healthy diet, exercising regularly, and avoiding exposure to toxins. By reducing inflammation, you may be able to improve symptoms of ADHD.

ANTI-INFLAMMATORY DIET

Are you looking for the next best diet trend? If yes, you're lucky - the latest diet includes anti-inflammatory foods. That's right, folks - food is the new medicine. But before you run to your kitchen and start stocking up on turmeric and ginger, you should know a few things about this diet trend. Here's what you need to know about anti-inflammatory foods.

There is a lot of buzz around omega-3 fatty acids for a good reason. These essential fats are found in many foods we commonly eat, including fish, nuts, and certain seeds. In addition, omega-3 fatty acids have powerful anti-inflammatory properties [16]. By reducing inflammation throughout the body, omega-3 fatty acids can help combat many conditions and diseases, from chronic pain to heart disease and more.

Turmeric is a spice that has been commonly used in Indian cuisine and for centuries in traditional Chinese and Ayurvedic medicine. Turmeric contains a compound called curcumin, which has been shown to have anti-inflammatory effects.

When it comes to health and wellness, green tea is considered a true powerhouse. Made from the delicate leaves of the Camellia sinensis plant, green tea is packed with nutrients that can help to support all aspects of our bodies. It also contains a powerful compound called EGCG, which has been shown to have potent anti-inflammatory effects. So, whether you are trying to fight off colds or ease joint pain, adding a few cups of green tea to your daily routine is what you need.

Ginger is one of the most popular spices in the world, used in everything from Asian dishes to baked goods [13]. The compound found in ginger, known as gingerol, has been extensively studied and shown to have potent anti-inflammatory effects. So, whether you're seeking relief from pain or discomfort or want to take advantage of all the nutritional benefits ginger offers, adding this incredible spice to your diet is sure to provide multiple health benefits.

Garlic is an ingredient that is used in many different cuisines. But many people don't realize that garlic has much more to offer than its superb flavor. This humble ingredient contains a powerful compound called allicin. This compound is shown to have potent anti-inflammatory effects. It can help relieve pain and inflammation associated with arthritis and gout.

Dark chocolate is made from the cacao bean and contains a high percentage of cocoa solids. Dark chocolate contains compounds, such as flavonoids, that help to reduce inflammation in the body [14]. These compounds, known as flavonoids, are responsible for dark chocolate's bitter taste. But while the bitterness may not be to everyone's liking, the health benefits of dark chocolate are hard to ignore. So, if you're looking for a delicious way to reduce inflammation and improve your overall health, reach for some dark chocolate the next time you have a sweet tooth.

While anti-inflammatory foods are good for you, it is possible to overeat them. This may result in an upset stomach or diarrhea. So be sure to moderate your intake and enjoy these healthy foods in moderation.

These are just a few of the many foods that contain compounds that help to reduce inflammation in the body [13]. By incorporating these anti-inflammatory foods into your diet, you can help to improve your health and well-being. Therefore, do not wait any longer; start adding these delicious and healthy foods to your diet today.

The bottom line is that your diet, and the inflammation it causes, have significant effects on your health. Inflammation doesn't just cause joint pain and make you feel generally lousy – it also leads to developing severe diseases [4]. But don't worry! You don't have to give up all your favorite foods to reduce inflammation and improve your health. Plenty of delicious (and healthy) recipes will help you get started on the road to better health.

Part II

CHAPTER 4

Nerves of the Body

Nerves are one of the most important and often overlooked body parts. They are responsible for transmitting messages, including sensory and motor messages, between the brain and the rest of the body. Unfortunately, nerves can be easily damaged or inflamed, leading to various problems.

Most people don't know much about nerves except that they sometimes get "pinched." This can lead to tingling, pain, or numbness in various body parts. In some cases, nerve damage is permanent. In others, it may be reversible with treatment. When nerves are damaged, they may lose contact with their target organs, hence, the passage of signals from the brain to the organs becomes impaired.

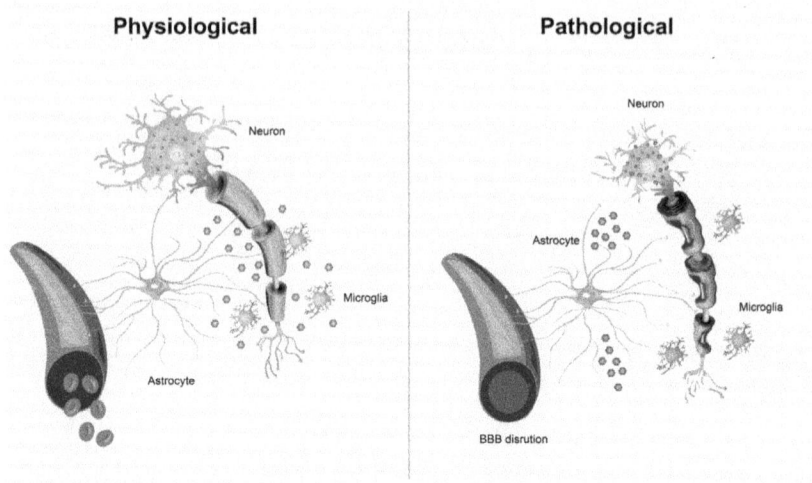

Figure 4: Nervous system

THE NERVOUS SYSTEM

The nervous system is composed of various cells, including neurons and glial cells. Neurons are the "thinking" and working cells of the nervous system. They send and receive electrical signals that allow the brain to communicate with the rest of the body (figure 4). Glial cells provide support, nutrition, and protection to the neurons.

The central and peripheral nervous systems are two parts of the nervous system. The brain and spinal cord are components of the central nervous system. The brain is the nerve control center for the neurological system. Signals from the senses are received through sensory neurons, while the signals to muscles and glands are sent out through motor neurons (in a hurry). A long, thin bundle of nerves known as the spinal cord, extends from the brain down to your lower back. It transmits information between the brain and other parts of your body.

The peripheral nervous system consists of all the nerves that branch off the spinal cord [27]. These nerves extend to every body part below the neck, including the arms, legs, and internal organs. The peripheral nervous system can be further divided into somatic and autonomic nervous systems.

The somatic nervous system controls the movement of voluntary muscles, such as those in the arms and legs. Conversely, the autonomic nervous system controls involuntary muscles in the heart, lungs, and digestive systems.

Nerves are a collection of neurons and supporting cells and are responsible for transmitting electrical signals between the body and the brain. The neurons are divided into a cell body and branching fibers called dendrites and axons. Dendrites do receive signals from other neurons and pass them on to the cell body. The cell body sends the signal down the axon to the next neuron.

Nerves are an essential part of the body, but they are also delicate. Nerve damage can occur from various causes, including physical trauma, infections, and exposure to certain toxins. When nerves are damaged, the result can be pain, weakness, paralysis, or even death.

TYPES OF NERVES

Ever wonder how your brain realizes when your hand is too close to a hot stove? Or how do your lungs know to keep breathing air even when you are asleep? It is all thanks to your efficient nervous system. This unique system comprises nerves, classified according to their function, structure, and location (figure 5).

Sensory nerves: relay information from the body to the brain. That is how you know when something is hot, cold, sharp, etc. These nerves are located in the skin, muscles, joints, and internal organs. They have a special coating that protects them from damage.

Motor nerves: send information from the brain to the muscles so we can perform basic tasks like picking up a pencil or taking a step. Unfortunately, these nerves are unprotected in the joints and muscles, making them highly vulnerable to injury.

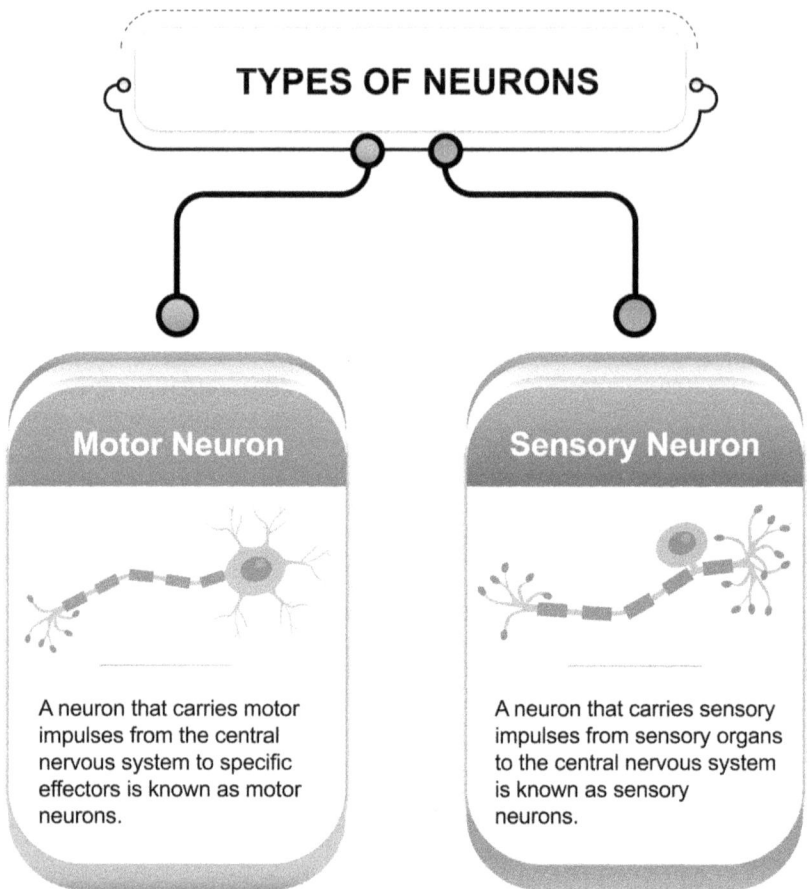

Figure 5: Types of neurons

Autonomic nerves regulate involuntary functions such as heart rate and blood pressure. These functions occur automatically without our realization. For example, as you read this passage, you don't realize that your heart is beating and the muscles in your stomach are contracting.

The autonomic nervous system is further divided into two parts: the sympathetic and the parasympathetic nervous system. The sympathetic nervous system refers to arousal (i.e. "fight or flight"), while the parasympathetic nervous system acts in opposition to it by promoting relaxation (or "rest and digest"). Both systems work together to keep the body in balance. The nerves controlling these two systems are located in the heart, blood vessels, smooth muscles, glands, and internal organs.

There you have it—a brief overview of the three types of nerves and what they do. Next time you accidentally stub your toe or have a close call with a hot stove, let's be grateful for your sensory nerves. Similarly, the next time you give someone a high five or take a step forward, let's be thankful for your motor nerves. Finally, let's be grateful for your autonomic nerves every time your heart beats, or you take a deep breath. These are functions that occur automatically without you even having to think about them. That is to say, we often take our nervous system for granted, which is impressive.

THE MAJOR INNERVATIONS OF THE BODY

The major innervations of the body originate in the brain and spinal cord. These include the sensory and motor systems, with specific function which helps to control all aspects of bodily function.

The spinal cord is the primary pathway for carrying information to and from the brain. It is made up of many nerves that branch off to innervate different parts of the body. The brainstem is located at the base of the brain and controls the body's automatic functions, such as heart rate and breathing.

The sympathetic nervous system is activated in response to stress and danger. It prepares the body for "fight or flight" by increasing heart rate and blood pressure. The parasympathetic nervous system has the opposite effect; it slows down the heart rate, reduces blood pressure and promotes digestion.

The enteric nervous system is a network of nerves that controls the digestive system. It is located in the gut walls and is responsible for many functions, such as digestion, absorption, and elimination.

All these innervations work together to keep the body functioning correctly. Without them, we would be unable to move, feel sensations, or digest food. So, next time you think about your nervous system, remember how magnificent your brains are and you might want to stop underestimating them.

FUNCTIONS OF THE NERVES

Did you know that the human body has approximately forty-five miles of nerves? That is many nerves. But what exactly do nerves do? Nerves help us see, hear, smell, taste, touch, and feel pain. Moreover, nerves help us maintain our balance and walk upright. In short, without nerves, we would not be able to live. Let's take a more in-depth look at each of these functions.

Nerves play a critical role in sight. Without them, we would not be able to see. Two nerve cells are responsible for your sight—rods and cones. Rods are responsible for black-and-white vision, while cones are responsible for color vision. Both nerve cells send electrical impulses from the back of the eyes to the brain through optic nerves, which are translated into images.

Nerve cells are responsible for our hearing. These nerve cells, called hair cells, have tiny hairs located in the inner ear. Hair cells translate sound waves into electrical impulses sent to the brain, where they are interpreted as sounds with specific meanings.

The nose can smell because of nerves. There are special cells in the nose that are called olfactory receptors. These cells send electrical impulses to the brain. The brain turns these impulses into smells.

Similar to smell, taste is also made possible by nerve cells. These cells called receptors, are located on the tongue and send electrical signals to the brain, which are translated into tastes. Have you ever stubbed your toe or burned yourself on a hot stove? If so, then you have your nerve cells to thank for that painful experience! That's because these nerve cells in the skin send electrical signals from the injury site to the brain, which are then translated into pain.

As you can see, there are many different functions of nerves in the human body. We rely on them every day— sometimes without even realizing it. So next time you stub your toe or take a bite of your favorite food, thank your nerves for making it all possible to sense or feel these moments.

NEUROPATHY

Neuropathy is a term used to describe a wide variety of disease conditions that affect the nervous system. Neuropathy can be caused by injury, disease, or even exposure to certain toxins. When nerve cells are damaged, they cannot correctly send electrical signals, leading to the development of different symptoms, such as numbness, tingling, pain, and weakness. Neuropathy is a serious condition that can significantly reduce the quality of life.

There are many different causes of neuropathy. One of the most common causes is diabetes mellitus. When blood sugar levels in the blood are high, it can damage nerve cells. Other common causes include alcoholism, certain medications, and vitamin deficiencies. In some cases, the cause of neuropathy is unknown.

Various treatments for neuropathy exist. The most common treatments include medications, surgery, and physical therapy. Medications can be used to help reduce pain and inflammation. Surgery may be necessary to repair damaged nerve cells. Physical therapy can help to improve the strength and mobility of muscles and joints. In some cases, lifestyle changes such as changes in diet or exercise may also be recommended.

Some neuropathy prevention methods are available. These include optimal control of blood sugar levels in patients with diabetes mellitus. Other lifestyle changes that may be helpful include eating a healthy diet, maintaining a healthy weight, and exercising regularly. If you are taking any medications associated with neuropathy, be sure to talk to your doctor about possible alternatives.

THE DOMINO EFFECT OF INFLAMMATION

We all know what it feels like to have a cold or the flu. We get a runny nose, our throat starts hurting, and we feel awful. But have you ever wondered why we think this way? It turns out that inflammation plays a significant role in these symptoms.

In some cases, the consequences of inflammation can be beneficial. For example, suppose you twist your ankle. In that case, the inflammation caused by the injury will help to protect the area and promote healing. However, in other cases, chronic inflammation can lead to health problems such as heart disease and arthritis [2]. The early parts of this chapter gave a detailed description of inflammation and its molecular mediators. Here, we will discuss the effects of inflammation on nervous systems.

INFLAMMATION OF THE SPINAL NERVES

As you read this, inflammation is silently raging inside your body. It's an ordinary and necessary process that helps fight infection and heals injuries [4]. But sometimes, for reasons we still don't fully understand, inflammation can spin out of control. As a result, the immune system starts attacking the body's tissues, leading to many health problems.

One of the organs most affected by uncontrolled inflammation is the spinal cord. This is because spinal nerves are specifically susceptible to inflammatory molecules called cytokines. Cytokines can cause nerve cells to die, leading to reduced function or even paralysis. There are three main ways in which inflammation can damage spinal nerves:

By damaging the myelin sheath- The myelin sheath is a protective layer surrounding neurons. It helps them to function correctly by keeping electrical impulses moving along their length. When the myelin sheath becomes damaged, it can cause movement, sensation, and cognition problems.

By damaging the actual nerve cells- Inflammation can also damage nerve cells directly. This can lead to loss of function or even death of the cells.

By causing gene expression changes [28], this is a severe side effect of inflammation. Once the damage has been done, it can be challenging to reverse. In addition, the changes in gene expression can cause cells to function differently than before the inflammation occurred. This can lead to long-term problems such as paralysis of limbs or loss of sensation.

It is called radiculopathy, when the spinal nerves become inflamed [29]. This condition can be excruciating and debilitating. In addition, the inflammation can damage the nerve cells, leading to a wide range of potential health problems. Radiculopathies can be due to different conditions, such as herniated discs, spinal stenosis, and degenerative disc disease. Inflammation can also be caused by injuries, infections, and autoimmune diseases.

The most common symptom of radiculopathy is pain, which can be mild or severe and may radiate from the spine to the arms or legs. Other symptoms include numbness, tingling, muscle weakness, and the problem with bowel or bladder control.

Radiculopathy can make it difficult to perform everyday activities like walking, sitting, and standing. It can also interfere with your ability to work or participate in leisure activities. In severe cases, radiculopathy can cause functional dependency and progressive paralysis.

No matter the cause, inflammation of the spinal nerves is a severe condition that requires prompt treatment. If left untreated, it can lead to permanent nerve damage and disability.

CHAPTER 5

The General Scheme of the Spinal Nerves

They are classified into, cervical, thoracic, lumber, sacral and coccygeal, each of which carries specific nerves to specific organs. The nerves originating from the spine to the organs are delicate. For example, when the cervical nerves (C1-C4) innervating the intracranial blood vessels are inflamed, migraine, headache or dizziness are the possible symptoms you could experience.

CERVICAL NERVES C1-C4

The cervical nerves are a group of spinal nerves that originate in the neck and travel down to the arms and hands. These are the uppermost spinal nerves and are distally followed by thoracic, lumbar, sacral, and coccygeal nerves (figure 6).

SPINAL NERVES INNERVATE EVERY ORGAN; BLOCKAGE OR INFLAMMATION OF THE NERVES AFFECT THE ORGANS AND THEY MANIFEST POSSIBLE SYMPTOMS

Nerve root	Organs	Possible symptoms
C1	1 Eyes	Vision problems
C2	2 Intracranial Blood vessels	Migraine, headache, dizziness
C2	3 Lacrimal gland	Sinus problems, runny nose, sore throat, cough, croup
C3	4 Parotid gland	Allergies
C4	5 Neck muscles	Stiff neck
C5	5 Neck muscles	Stiff neck
C6	6 Arms	Arm pain
C6	7 Wrists, hands, fingers	Hand and finger numbness
C7	8 Lungs	Asthma
C8	9 Chest	Heart conditions
T1	10 Arms	Wrists, hands, fingers numbness or pain
T2	11 Lungs	Congestion
T3	12 Larynx, Trachea	Difficulty breathing, asthma
T4	13 Heart	High blood pressure, heart conditions
T5		
T6	14 Gall bladder, liver	Gall bladder conditions, jaundice, liver conditions
T7	15 Stomach	Stomach problems, ulcers, gastritis
T8	16 Spleen	Jaundice
T9	17 Kidneys	Kidney problems
T10		
T11	23 Small intestine, colon	Intestinal obstruction, ulcers, etc
T12	24 Uterus	Menstrual problems
L1	18 Large intestine	Constipation, colitis, diarrhea
L2	19 Reproductive organs	Menstrual problems
L3	20 Legs	Pin and numbness of legs
L4	21 Buttocks	Low back pain
L5		
S		
A	19 Reproductive organs	Menstrual problems
C	20 Legs, ankles, feet, toes	Pain or numbness in legs
R	21 Buttocks	Lower back pain, leg numbness
A	22 Bladder	Bladder problems
L		

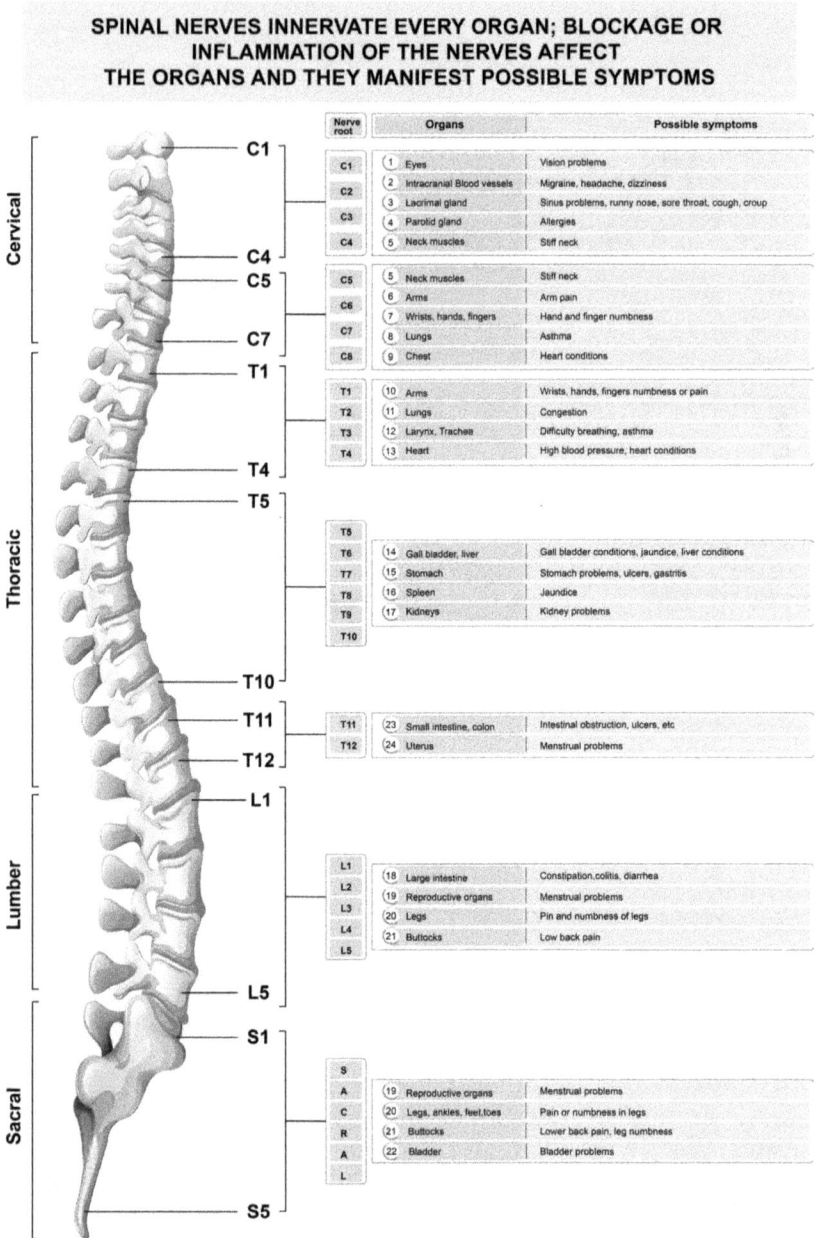

Figure 6: The general scheme of the spinal nerves.

The cervical nerves are responsible for carrying messages from the brain to the muscles, skin, and other tissues. In addition, they carry the sensory messages from the skin and internal organs to the brain. The cervical nerves are composed of eight pairs of nerves numbered C1 through C8 [27]. The first four pairs (C1-C4) originate in the neck, and the last four pairs (C5-C8) develop in the chest.

Each cervical nerve is responsible for innervating different parts of the body. For example, C1-C3 (the first three cervical nerves) help control the head and neck, while C4 helps control upward shoulder movements. Additionally, C4 (along with C3 and C5) helps power the diaphragm— the sheet of muscle stretching to the rib cage's bottom for breathing [30].

The cervical nerves (C1-C4) are responsible for sensation in the upper head, side of the face, and back of the head. C1 doesn't have a dermatome, or the area of the skin supplied by a single nerve, while C2 and C3 handle trends for the upper part of the head and side of the face, respectively. Finally, C4 covers aspects of the arms' neck, shoulders, and upper leg.

Cervical nerves C1-C4 play an essential role in the function of the eyes and glands. Both C1 and C2 supply the nerves that control eye movements. C3 innervates the trigeminal nerve, which controls sensation in the face. It supplies parasympathetic fibers to the lacrimal gland (which produces tears). Finally, C4 innervates the facial nerve, which controls facial muscles and provides parasympathetic fibers to the parotid gland (which produces saliva).

Cervical nerves C1-C4 can become inflamed for various reasons, including injury, infection, and exposure to toxins. When these nerves are inflamed, it can cause several symptoms, including pain, numbness, tingling, weakness, and problems with coordination and balance [29].

The most common symptom of inflammation of the cervical nerves is pain, which can range from mild to severe, and may radiate down into the arms and hands.

The pain may be constant or intermittent and may get worse with specific activities, such as moving the neck or head. The pain may also spread from the upper neck into the back of the head, causing a cervicogenic headache or migraine.

Numbness and tingling are other common symptoms of cervical nerve inflammation. This numbness and tingling may be felt in the arms, hands, fingers, or legs as well as in the face, scalp, or neck.

Weakness is another common symptom of nerve damage. This is due to injury or paralysis of muscles. The weakness can make it difficult to perform activities that require using the arm or hand, such as writing, brushing teeth, or combing hair. Problems with coordination and balance can also occur when the cervical nerves are inflamed. This can make it difficult to walk or stand and may cause falls.

If the phrenic nerve is damaged, it may cause difficulty or an inability to breathe. This is because the phrenic nerve helps control the diaphragm, the primary muscle of breathing, which may not work correctly when damaged. This can lead to several problems, such as difficulty breathing, shortness of breath, and even respiratory failure.

Symptoms of cervical nerve inflammation can also include sinus issues, a cough, allergies, and a sore throat. If you are experiencing any of these symptoms, you must see a doctor for diagnosis and treatment.

The symptoms of inflammation of the cervical nerves C1-C4 can vary in severity depending on the underlying cause. In some cases, the symptoms may be so mild that they go unnoticed. In other cases, the symptoms can be severe and debilitating.

CERVICAL NERVES C5-C8

Cervical nerves (C5-C8 vertebrae) control the muscles and sensations in your neck, shoulders, arms, and hands. They originate in the cervical spine, which comprises the

C5-C8 vertebrae. Damage to these nerves can cause various symptoms, depending on the location and degree of injury.

The C5 is primarily responsible for controlling the outer contours of the shoulders and upper arms. It also helps in bending and rotating the elbows. The C6 controls the allowed flexing or bending of the wrist.

C7 controls the triceps muscle on the back of the forearm, which is involved in straightening the elbow. Finally, C8 is instrumental in controlling various functions of your hands, particularly finger flexion (or handgrip). With so much important work going on here, it's easy to see why these nerves are essential for staying active and keeping yourself in top form.

The cervical nerves (C5-C8 vertebrae) can become inflamed for several reasons, such as infection, injury, or compression. This may cause various symptoms, including neck pain, arm pain, tingling or numbness in the hands or arms, and weakness in the arms or hands. This is because these nerves control the muscles and sensations in these body areas.

You must immediately see a doctor if you're experiencing any of these symptoms. Treatment will depend on the underlying cause but may include rest, ice, heat, physical therapy, or medication. In addition, surgery may sometimes be necessary to relieve pressure on the nerves or repair the damage.

THORACIC NERVES T1-T4

The thoracic nerves are a group of twelve nerves that originate in the thoracic part of the spinal cord [29]. These nerves innervate the chest, back, and abdomen muscles and skin. The thoracic nerves are divided into the posterior (dorsal) thoracic and anterior (ventral) thoracic nerves.

Thoracic nerves T1-T4 innervate the chest, back, and abdominal muscles and skin. They also innervate the esophagus, heart, lungs, chest, and trachea. This allows these organs to function correctly and communicate with the brain and spinal cord to ensure optimal function.

T1 and T2 are two essential thoracic nerves that provide critical input to the chest wall and the arm and hand. While T1 acts mainly as part of the brachial plexus, a network of nerves controlling the arm, T2 feeds into nerves that go into the top of the chest, arm, and hand [30]. In addition, the throat and glands within each lung also receive signals from these powerful nerves, allowing them to function appropriately during respiration.

Meanwhile, T3 and T4 play an essential role in facilitating breathing. These nerves feed directly into the chest wall, relaying signals that allow for proper expansion and contraction of the lungs during each breath. Through their intricate network of connections, these three vital nerves help keep us alive and thriving daily [31].

Common injuries to the thoracic nerves include:
• Compression (such as from a herniated disc of the vertebra).

- Trauma (such as from a car accident).
- Surgery (such as thoracotomy).

These injuries can cause paralysis, loss of sensation, and other problems associated with nerve injury.

The thoracic nerves are vital for adequately functioning several organs in the chest and abdomen [27]. These nerves' primary function is to send signals between the brain and these organs, ensuring that breathing and blood pressure are appropriately regulated. However, when these nerves become inflamed, they can cause highly unpleasant symptoms, including congestion, high blood pressure, and breathing difficulties.

Because of the importance of these nerves for our overall health and well-being, we must take steps to prevent inflammation in the thoracic area. Focusing on maintaining a healthy lifestyle and paying attention to signs of inflammation or poor health can help keep our thoracic nerves functioning at total capacity, allowing us to lead happier and healthier lives.

THORACIC NERVES T5-T10

When it comes to nerves, the T5-T8 are among the most important. These nerves are responsible for controlling the movements of abdominal muscles [27]. Thus, any pain symptoms in this area will be expressed through issues with the abdomen. For example, those who experience problems with digestion, such as ulcers or heartburn, may be dealing with some form of injury or strain on the T5 and T6 nerves. T5 also regulates the function of the liver.

And if that isn't bad enough, further injuries to the T7 and T8 nerves can have even more severe consequences, leading to a host of other problems, including fatigue, anemia, weak circulation, a weakened immune system, and low blood pressure. Considering all this, taking care of your T5-T8 nerves is essential for maintaining overall health and well-being.

T10 is a crucial nerve responsible for innervating the lower abdomen muscles. Every time you bend down to tie your shoes or stand up from sitting on the floor, you rely on

T10 to fire up and contract those all-important abdominal muscles. T10 also plays a vital role in moving your legs and trunk when you walk. It also sends some branches to the kidneys.

When it comes to disability, the extent of the damage is often determined by the amount of damage done to the T10 vertebra. In cases with only mild and partial injury to this vertebra, a patient may only experience weakness, numbness, loss of muscle control, or lack of use of only one side of the lower body.

However, if there is complete damage to this area - in other words, if the T10 vertebra has sustained destruction - then the likelihood that the patient loses all motor function in the lower body (including their legs) could be extremely high. This condition, termed paraplegia, is one of the most severe disabilities a person can experience. Fortunately, with proper care and rehabilitation techniques, many patients with moderate or severe disabilities can fully recover and regain at least some degree of mobility of the affected limbs.

THORACIC NERVE T11

The T11 nerve controls many vital areas and functions of our bodies. Located at the lower back, near the base of the spine, this robust bundle of nerves has many responsibilities that directly impact our health and well-being [32]. For example, the kidneys, ureters, small intestines, colon, and uterus are all supplied by the T11 nerve. All these organs play a critical role in our overall health by ensuring that waste materials are filtered out from our bloodstream and effectively excreted by the kidneys. Additionally, by regulating intestinal function, this nerve helps to keep us regular and prevent problems like constipation or bloating.

The sensory supply of the T11 nerve is located on the midclavicular line, at the horizontal level midway between the level of the umbilicus and the inguinal ligament; this region contains several interconnected nerves that carry sensations gathered from various parts of the body. These sensations are then sent to multiple brain parts, processed, and interpreted by our subconscious minds.

When dealing with a T11 injury, it is essential to understand the signs that this type of injury will present. Severe back and leg pain are key indicators that the nerves in the T11 vertebrae may have been damaged or otherwise impacted. In addition, patients with this injury may also experience weakness and numbness in these areas and other related symptoms like kidney or intestinal issues. Notice these symptoms after an accident or injury. You must get medical help immediately to start addressing and managing your injuries. You can fully recover from a T11 injury and regain your health and well-being with proper treatment and care.

THORACIC NERVE T12

The thoracic nerve plays a critical role in several body functions. For example, this powerful nerve innervates the uterus and colon, helping to control contractions and digestion. It also sends signals to the muscles of our buttocks and small intestine, allowing us to move and process food efficiently. However, one of these strong nerves' most essential jobs is regulating lymph circulation. The lymphatic system functions in our bodies, filtering toxins and waste products while fighting off infections. And it is the thoracic nerve that provides this system with much-needed energy and stimulation, ensuring that our immune systems are running at peak performance.

When the T12 region develops inflammation, it can cause a wide range of uncomfortable and potentially dangerous symptoms. These may include difficulty breathing as air passages become restricted due to swelling in the area. In addition, bowel and bladder dysfunction is expected, as the nerves that regulate these functions are often affected by inflammation of the T12.

Some people also experience ulcers in the back, which may require medication or surgical intervention. Moreover, those with T12 inflammation may also develop kidney problems, such as blood in the urine or reduced urine output. However, most people can effectively manage their T12 inflammation and restore their quality of life through careful management and treatment by a skilled medical professional.

LUMBER NERVES L1-L5

The lumber nerves innervate the large intestine, buttocks, reproductive organs, colon, thighs, knees, and leg [33]. These nerves originate in the spinal cord and run through the vertebrae in the lower back (lumbar region). There are five pairs of primary lumber nerves (L1-L5), each of which is responsible for innervating specific lower body parts [27].

An inflammation of the lumber nerve occurs when the nerves in your lower back become inflamed or irritated. This may occur due to poor posture or herniated discs. However, suppose you're dealing with chronic inflammation. In that case, you may find it challenging to perform even basic tasks like going to work or taking care of your family.

Suppose you are experiencing common symptoms of lumber nerve inflammation, such as constipation, gas, bloating, irritable bowel, menstrual problems, or back pain. In that case, you may be wondering what could be causing these troubling symptoms. In most cases, lumber nerve inflammation is caused by some underlying health condition, such as an infection or autoimmune disorder.

However, other factors, such as stress and poor diet, can also contribute to inflammation in the body. Suppose you are experiencing persistent issues with your lumber nerves and the accompanying symptoms, it may be essential to see a doctor for further assessment and treatment options.

SACRAL NERVES S1-S5

The sacral nerves are a group of nerves arising from the sacral plexus - a network of nerve fibers in the lower back [34]. There are five pairs of sacral nerves, numbered S1-S5 [35]. These nerves innervate the muscles and skin of the buttocks, and the various organs in the pelvic region, including the reproductive organs and bladder. The sacral nerves also carry sensations from the legs and feet.

The sacral nerves are essential in controlling several essential body functions related to reproduction, urination, and defecation. They also help prevent the muscles of the pelvis and legs. As a result, disorders of the sacral nerves can lead to a wide range of issues, including urinary and fecal incontinence, sexual dysfunction, and problems with movement.

Following inflammation of these nerves, symptoms varies greatly depending on which nerves are affected. For example, diarrhea and constipation are common signs of sacral nerve inflammation in S1 and S2. Further, sacral nerve inflammation in S3-S5 is often associated with cramping or menstrual problems in women. Additionally, individuals with sacral nerve inflammation may experience back pain or numbness in their legs.

In case of the development of diarrhea, back pain, or something else, it is vital to seek medical attention immediately. You can manage your condition and alleviate any discomfort you may be experiencing with proper treatment and care.

COCCYGEAL NERVES

Coccygeal nerves, also known as the tailbone nerves, are the smallest and final pair of spinal nerves [35]. They originate from a part of the spinal cord that many people do not know exists. They relay messages from our tailbone to the brain, sending signals about touch, temperature, pain, and pressure. This allows us to detect any damage or injury near our tailbone area to react quickly and ensure that we do not harm ourselves further.

In addition to their sensory functions, the coccygeal nerves also play critical roles in motor control. They act as connections between muscles in our lower back and pelvis for smooth movement throughout the day. Without these functions, we will develop weakness in our feet.

Coccydynia, more commonly known as inflammation of the coccyx, is a common condition that occurs due to several factors. However, the main culprit for many people is direct trauma to the tailbone, such as a fall or other impact injury. The surrounding tissue becomes inflamed and irritated, leading to pain and discomfort.

However, other underlying factors, such as nerve compression or bone spurs, may contribute to coccydynia in some cases. Regardless of the cause, however, rest and over-the-counter pain medications are typically recommended to help reduce inflammation and ease any associated discomfort.

In conclusion, nerves play a vital role in the body, controlling and regulating different functions. When these nerves become inflamed, it can cause pain and discomfort. There are many reasons why this inflammation may occur. Still, some of the most common include injuries, infections, or autoimmune diseases.

Injuries to the spinal cord can cause temporary or permanent damage, leading to paralysis or loss of sensation. Treatment for such injuries depends on the severity and may include surgery, medication, physical therapy, or rehabilitation [32, 36]. However, with proper care and treatment, many people with spinal cord injuries can lead entire and productive lives.

Final Remarks

Altogether, we summarize two important topics in this chapter. We discuss inflammation, which is the body's response to an injury or trauma. Short-term inflammation is critical for ensuring optimal repair and healing. However, chronic uncontrolled inflammation can lead to several diseases, including cancer, cardiovascular disorders, neurological diseases, and degenerative conditions. Inflammation is also a critical factor in ageing. We also discuss several foods and lifestyles, which can promote or prevent inflammation, and their roles in regulating health and disease.

Lastly, we discuss the nervous system and its critical role in controlling body functions. The nervous system consists of two types of neurons, including sensory and motor neurons. Sensory neurons carry sensations from the body to the brain, while motor neurons carry motor signals from the brain to the body. Motor signals can be somatic, meaning they go to skeletal muscle, and we can voluntarily control them, such as the movement of the arms. Motor signals can also be autonomic, which are outside our voluntary control, such as breathing, the beating of the heart, etc. We also discussed nerves originating from the spinal cord and carrying sensory and motor signals to different body parts. We have clarified how inflammation of nerves innervating these organs can produce notable symptoms. When you realize these symptoms, talk to your Physician. At this point, you could say, you are your own Physician first!

References

1. Lucas, L., A. Russell, and R. Keast, *Molecular mechanisms of inflammation. Anti-inflammatory benefits of virgin olive oil and the phenolic compound oleocanthal.* Curr Pharm Des, 2011. 17(8): p. 754-68.

2. Libby, P. and S. Kobold, *Inflammation: a common contributor to cancer, aging, and cardiovascular diseases-expanding the concept of cardio-oncology.* Cardiovasc Res, 2019. 115(5): p. 824-829.

3. Caruso, G., et al., *Inflammation as the Common Biological Link Between Depression and Cardiovascular Diseases: Can Carnosine Exert a Protective Role?* Curr Med Chem, 2020. 27(11): p. 1782-1800.

4. Liu, Y.Z., Y.X. Wang, and C.L. Jiang, *Inflammation: The Common Pathway of Stress-Related Diseases.* Front Hum Neurosci, 2017. 11: p. 316.

5. Decker, A., et al., *The assessment of stress, depression, and inflammation as a collective risk factor for periodontal diseases: a systematic review.* Clin Oral Investig, 2020. 24(1): p. 1-12.

6. Rocha, P.N., T.J. Plumb, and T.M. Coffman, *Eicosanoids: lipid mediators of inflammation in transplantation.* Springer Semin Immunopathol, 2003. 25(2): p. 215-27.

7. Yamaguchi, A., E. Botta, and M. Holinstat, *Eicosanoids in inflammation in the blood and the vessel.* Front Pharmacol, 2022. 13: p. 997403.

8. Antonova, M., et al., *Prostaglandins in migraine: update.* Curr Opin Neurol, 2013. 26(3): p. 269-75.

9. Xu, H., et al., *Network meta-analysis of migraine disorder treatment* by NSAIDs and triptans. J Headache Pain, 2016. 17(1): p. 113.

10. Umamaheswaran, S., et al., *Stress, inflammation, and eicosanoids: an emerging perspective.* Cancer Metastasis Rev, 2018. 37(2-3): p. 203-211.

11. Chen, K., et al., *Brain injury and inflammation genes common to a number of neurological diseases and the genes involved in the genesis of GABAnergic neurons are altered in monoamine oxidase B knockout mice.* Brain Res, 2022. 1774: p. 147724.

12. Gu, Y., et al., *High-Fat Diet-Induced Obesity Aggravates Food Allergy by Intestinal Barrier Destruction and Inflammation.* Int Arch Allergy Immunol, 2022. 183(1): p. 80-92.

13. Mayer, C. and J. Reuter, *Molecular Nutrition & Food Research - Functional Relevance of Dietetics and Its Impact on Gut Microbiome, Inflammation and Obesity.* Mol Nutr Food Res, 2022. 66(1): p. e2270003.

14. Mignogna, C., et al., *The inflammatory potential of the diet as a link between food processing and low-grade*

inflammation: An analysis on 21,315 participants to the Moli-sani study. Clin Nutr, 2022. 41(10): p. 2226-2234.

15. Luvian-Morales, J., et al., *Functional foods modulating inflammation and metabolism in chronic diseases: a systematic review.* Crit Rev Food Sci Nutr, 2022. 62(16): p. 4371-4392.

16. Bourre, J.M., *Effects of nutrients (in food) on the structure and function of the nervous system: update on dietary requirements for brain.* Part 2 : macronutrients. J Nutr Health Aging, 2006. 10(5): p. 386-99.

17. Strzelak, A., et al., *Tobacco Smoke Induces and Alters Immune Responses in the Lung Triggering Inflammation, Allergy, Asthma and Other Lung Diseases: A Mechanistic Review.* Int J Environ Res Public Health, 2018. 15(5).

18. Stolp, H.B. and K.M. Dziegielewska, *Review: Role of developmental inflammation and blood-brain barrier dysfunction in neurodevelopmental and*

neurodegenerative diseases. Neuropathol Appl Neurobiol, 2009. 35(2): p. 132-46.

19. Finelli, R., et al., *The impact of autoimmune systemic inflammation and associated medications on male reproductive health in patients with chronic rheumatological, dermatological, and gastroenterological diseases: A systematic review.* Am J Reprod Immunol, 2021. 85(5): p. e13389.

20. Saccaro, L.F., et al., *Inflammation, Anxiety, and Stress in Attention-Deficit/Hyperactivity Disorder.* Biomedicines, 2021. 9(10).

21. Litvack, M.L. and N. Palaniyar, *Review: Soluble innate immune pattern-recognition proteins for clearing dying cells and cellular components: implications on exacerbating or resolving inflammation.* Innate Immun, 2010. 16(3): p. 191-200.

22. Nikoopour, E., J.A. Schwartz, and B. Singh, *Therapeutic benefits of regulating inflammation in autoimmunity.* Inflamm Allergy Drug Targets, 2008. 7(3): p. 203-10.

23. Leffa, D.T., et al., *Attention-deficit/hyperactivity disorder has a state-dependent association with asthma: The role of systemic inflammation in a population-based birth cohort followed from childhood to adulthood.* Brain Behav Immun, 2021. 97: p. 239-249.

24. Manolis, A.S. and A.G. Tzioufas, *Cardio-Rheumatology: Cardiovascular Complications in Systemic Autoimmune Rheumatic Diseases / Is Inflammation the Common Link and Target?* Curr Vasc Pharmacol, 2020. 18(5): p. 425-430.

25. Namjoo, I., et al., *The Relationship Between Antioxidants and Inflammation in Children With Attention Deficit Hyperactivity Disorder.* Basic Clin Neurosci, 2020. 11(3): p. 313-321.

26. Alvarez-Arellano, L., et al., *Antioxidants as a Potential Target against Inflammation and Oxidative Stress in Attention-Deficit/Hyperactivity Disorder.* Antioxidants (Basel), 2020. 9(2).

27. Mainkar, O., et al., *Ultrasound-Guided Peripheral Nerve Stimulation of Cervical, Thoracic, and Lumbar Spinal Nerves for Dermatomal Pain: A Case Series.* Neuromodulation, 2021. 24(6): p. 1059-1066.

28. O'Connor, R.A. and S.M. *Anderton, Inflammation-associated genes: risks and benefits to Foxp3+ regulatory T-cell function.* Immunology, 2015. 146(2): p. 194-205.

29. Cummings, K.W., et al., *Cross-sectional Imaging Anatomy and Pathologic Conditions Affecting Thoracic Nerves.* Radiographics, 2017. 37(1): p. 73-92.

30. Guilherme, S. and L. Benigni, *Ultrasonographic anatomy of the brachial plexus and major nerves of*

the canine thoracic limb. Vet Radiol Ultrasound, 2008. 49(6): p. 577-83.

31. Loukas, M., et al., *A review of the thoracic splanchnic nerves and celiac ganglia*. Clin Anat, 2010. 23(5): p. 512-22.

32. Yang, H.J., et al., *Anatomy of thoracic splanchnic nerves for surgical resection*. Clin Anat, 2008. 21(2): p. 171-7.

33. Breemer, M.C., M.J.A. Malessy, and R.G.E. Notenboom, *Origin, branching pattern, foraminal and intraspinal distribution of the human lumbar sinuvertebral nerves*. Spine J, 2022. 22(3): p. 472-482.

34. Possover, M., V. Chiantera, and J. Baekelandt, *Anatomy of the Sacral Roots and the Pelvic Splanchnic Nerves in Women Using the LANN Technique*. Surg Laparosc Endosc Percutan Tech, 2007. 17(6): p. 508-10.

35. Jin, Z.W., et al., Median Sacral Artery, *Sympathetic Nerves, and the Coccygeal Body: A Study Using Serial Sections of Human Embryos and Fetuses.* Anat Rec (Hoboken), 2016. 299(7): p. 819-27.

36. Iida, T., et al., *Sacral defect reconstruction using a sensate superior gluteal artery perforator flap based on the superior cluneal nerves: A report of two cases.* Microsurgery, 2021. 41(5): p. 468-472.

www.ingramcontent.com/pod-product-compliance
Lightning Source LLC
Chambersburg PA
CBHW052118030426

42335CB00025B/3046